MW00443584

The Glow-15 Diet Cookbook

A lifestyle plan that will make you lose weight, look and feel younger in just 15 days.

By

Laura Williams

Disclaimer:

The information provided in this book is designed to provide helpful information on the subjects discussed. The publisher and author are not responsible for any specific health or allergy needs that may require medical supervision and are not liable for any damages or negative consequences from any treatment, action, application or preparation, to any person reading or following the information in this book.

Table of Contents

INTRODUCTION:

Eating healthy makes you glow, lose weight and live healthy

I want you to know that eating right is a lifestyle and with anything in life we hit bumps in the road. In the beginning it may be tough to keep up, but NEVER give up, keep paddling.

Healthy eating and exercising holds many benefits which are as follows; it makes you feel better, keep you mentally alert, build a stronger immune system, and help you maintain a healthy weight.

If you looking lose a significant amount of weight knows that healthy eating is a major factor in the process. Furthermore, there are certain diseases where healthy eating is a must to stay alive such as heart disease, cancer, diabetes, Crohn's disease, and arthritis are a few diseases that people must follow a healthy diet.

However, eating the right combination of superfoods, such as whole grains, fresh produce, lean protein, and low-fat dairy will give your body the energy it needs and protect you from all the chronic diseases. Giving your fitness routines the time and dedication needed will also help fasten your fitness results.

In addition, doing the same workout or eating the same meal might be convenient, but for the results you want, it's good to spice up your food regimen and try different fitness activities. If you either trying to lose weight, lower your stress level, or looking for new ways to eat healthy and glow, each day is a new day to tackle your goals.

If you master the power of will and have a relentless attitude, I promise you will see many rewards. I advise you always hold yourself accountable to the best of your ability and you will never have any regrets.

Remember your body does not have the ability to turn garbage into a high-quality product. Your cells, bones, muscles, skin, etc. are built by the food that you supply. So I urge you to choose wisely. However, if you treat your body right it will treat you right. Time tells, in the long run your body will either be your best friend or your own worst enemy. The decision is all up to you to make!

Finally, try to get control of your eating this year, – so you can get control over your body

The Glow 15 recipes to help you Lose Weight, Revitalize Your Skin, and Invigorate Your Life

Stuffed Mushrooms

INGREDIENTS:

Low-fat (100g) ricotta cheese

Boneless leg ham (about 30g)

20g Diced red capsicum

Three medium (about 250g) Portobello mushrooms

Low fat (about 40g) grated cheddar cheese

1/4 cup Chopped parsley

Directions:

1. Meanwhile, you heat oven to 180 degrees Celsius.
2. After which you remove the stems from the mushrooms and dice them; finely cut the ham.
3. After that, you combine the capsicum, ricotta cheese ham, parsley, and diced mushroom stems in a bowl and mix well
4. Then you spoon the above mixture into the inverted mushrooms.
5. At this point, you sprinkle with the grated cheese.
6. Finally, you cook in pre-heated oven still at 180 degrees Celsius for 20 minutes.

Mushroom Delight

Ingredients:

75g green beans (chopped)

1 spring of onion

5g garlic (minced)

10g of grated cheese

260g Portobello mushrooms (chopped)

About 50g grated zucchini

2 (about 90g each) large eggs

10g of wholegrain mustard

Directions:

1. First, you mix all ingredients except cheese and eggs in a non-stick frying pan and cook for about 5 to 10 minutes on high heat (NOTE: no oil is needed as the mushrooms will lose water which will flow into the frying pan).
2. After which you add eggs and cook for a further 1-2 minutes
3. Then you remove from heat and serve with cheese sprinkled on top.

Low-Calorie Carbonara

Ingredients:

About 150mls of low-fat thickened cream

Rice bran cooking spray (to cook the bacon).

About 250g packet of Slender noodles

Bacon (with the fat removed)

Parmesan cheese (to taste)

Directions:

1. First, you cut the bacon into small pieces and fry it in cooking spray or a very small amount of cooking oil.
2. After which you add thickened cream and leave to boil for a couple of minutes to make sauce.
3. After that, you remove sauce from heat and prepare noodles as per instructions on packet.
4. Then you add sauce to noodles and mix together thoroughly.
5. At this point, you add parmesan cheese to taste but be sure to measure how much you're adding so you can work out how many calories are in it.
6. This is when you cook noodles as per instructions on packet

Clear Mushroom Soup

Ingredients:

2 cloves garlic.

2 spring onions (thin sliced).

Thick cut Portobello, Field and Shitake mushrooms (NOTE: enough to satisfy).

5 shallots (cut).

2 small chillis.

Directions:

1. First, you lightly fry in deep pot with a tiny spray of oil.
2. After which you add 500 ml of either Chicken, Beef or better still Vegetable stock; ground pepper to taste.
3. Then you bring to boil, then simmer for about 20 mins or as desired.

NOTE: this meal is usually around 100 calories depending on quantities.

Home-made coconut ice-cream

Yields: As much as you want to make

Equipment: Nutri-bullet

Ingredients

Vanilla essence (to taste, it is optional)

Stevia, natural sweetener (to taste, it is optional)

Coconut cream, as much as you like (you may use 'light' or low-fat for a lower calorie count)

Directions:

1. First, you place the coconut cream in the fridge overnight then in the freezer for an hour prior to making the ice-cream.

(**NOTE:** If it hasn't been in the fridge first, I suggest you leave it in the freezer for two hours).

2. After which you place the chilled/semi-frozen coconut cream and sweetener (optional) in the nutri-bullet and blast until the coconut cream goes solid enough that it no longer moves around in the nutri-bullet.
3. Then you serve and enjoy straight away before it melts. (**NOTE:** do not place it in the freezer as it will go as hard as ice).

Scrambled eggs with halloumi cheese

Ingredients

4 oz. bacon (diced)

2 scallions

8 tablespoons of pitted olives

Salt and pepper

4 eggs

3 oz. halloumi cheese (diced)

8 tablespoons of fresh parsley (chopped)

2 tablespoons of olive oil

Directions:

1. First, you dice halloumi cheese and bacon.
2. After which you heat olive oil on medium-high in a frying pan and fry halloumi, scallions and bacon until nicely browned.
3. After that, you whisk together eggs, parsley, salt and pepper.
4. Then you pour the egg mixture into the frying pan over the bacon and cheese.
5. At this point, you lower the heat, add the olives, and stir for a couple of minutes.
6. Finally, you serve with or without a salad.

NOTE:

Feel free to exclude the bacon if you are a vegetarian. You may also substitute the halloumi cheese with a different cheese such as mozzarella or feta and make sure you do not fry it; just add it in towards the end.

Low-carb blueberry smoothie

Ingredients

½ cup of fresh blueberries (fresh or frozen)

½ teaspoon of vanilla extract

14 oz. coconut milk

1 tablespoon of lemon juice

Directions:

1. First, you place all ingredients in the blender and mix until smooth.
2. After which you use a canned coconut milk (drain off the liquid) makes a creamier, more satisfying smoothie.
3. Then you taste, and add more lemon juice if desired.

NOTE:

I suggest you add 1 tablespoon of coconut oil or any other healthful oil for a more filling smoothie. Feel free to substitute the coconut milk for 1¼ cups Greek yogurt if you prefer a dairy-based smoothie. If so, I suggest you add a little water for a more liquid consistency.

Glow Deviled eggs

Ingredients

> 1 teaspoon of Tabasco
>
> 1 pinch of herbal salt
>
> Fresh Dill
>
> 4 hard-boiled eggs
>
> 4 tablespoons of mayonnaise
>
> 8 cooked and peeled shrimp (or better still a strips of smoked salmon)

Directions:

1. First, you split the eggs in half and scoop out the yolks.
2. After which you place the egg whites on a plate.
3. After that, you mash the yolks with a fork and stir in Tabasco, herbal salt and homemade mayonnaise.
4. Then you put the mayonnaise in the egg whites and top with a shrimp on each, or a piece of smoked salmon.
5. Finally, you decorate with dill.

NOTE:

I suggest you add capers for a bit of additional bit of salty and vinegary goodness.

Mexican scrambled eggs

Ingredients

1 scallion

1 tomato (finely chopped)

Salt and pepper

6 eggs

2 pickled jalapeños (finely chopped)

3 oz. shredded cheese

2 tablespoons of butter (for frying)

Directions:

1. First, you finely chop the scallions, jalapeños and tomatoes.
2. After which you fry in butter for about 3 minutes on medium heat.
3. After that, you beat in the eggs and pour into the pan.
4. Finally, you scramble for about 2 minutes and then add the cheese and seasoning.
5. Make sure you serve with avocado, crisp lettuce and dressing to add even more excitement to this zesty meal.

Egg muffins

Ingredients

1 scallion (finely chopped)

3 oz. of shredded cheese

Salt and pepper

6 eggs

5 oz. of air-dried chorizo or better still salami or cooked bacon

1 tablespoon of red pesto or green pesto (it is optional)

Directions:

1. Meanwhile, you heat the oven to 350°F (175°C).
2. After which you chop scallions and meat.
3. After that, you whisk the eggs together with seasoning and pesto.
4. Then you add the cheese and stir.
5. Furthermore, you place the batter in muffin forms and add bacon, chorizo or salami.
6. Finally, you bake for about 15–20 minutes, depending on the size of the muffin forms.

NOTE:

This recipe is perfect for a lunchbox; my kids love these cheesy muffins.

Browned butter asparagus with creamy eggs

Ingredients

4 eggs

8 tablespoons of sour cream

Cayenne pepper

1 tablespoon of olive oil

5 oz. of butter

3 oz. of grated parmesan cheese

Salt

1½ lbs. of green asparagus

1½ tablespoons of lemon juice

Directions:

1. First, you melt the butter over medium heat and add the eggs.
2. After which you stir until scrambled; cook through, but do not overcook the eggs.
3. After that, you spoon the hot eggs into a blender.
4. Then you add the cheese and sour cream and blend until smooth and creamy.
5. At this point, you add salt and cayenne pepper to taste.
6. Furthermore, you roast the asparagus in olive oil over medium heat in a large frying pan.

7. After that, you add salt and pepper, remove from frying pan for now, and set aside.
8. Then you sauté the butter in the frying pan until it is golden brown and has a nutty smell.
9. This is when you remove from heat, let cool, and add the lemon juice.
10. Finally, you put the asparagus back into the frying pan and stir together with the butter until it gets hot.
11. Make sure you serve the asparagus with the sautéed butter and the creamy eggs.

NOTE:

Remember, these creamy, cheesy eggs go with almost anything! I suggest you try them with fish, a nice steak, or other veggies.

Glow western omelet

Ingredients

2 tablespoons of heavy whipping cream (or better still sour cream)

3 oz. of shredded cheese

½ yellow onion (finely chopped)

5 oz. of smoked deli ham (diced)

6 eggs

Salt and pepper

2 oz. of butter

½ green bell pepper (finely chopped)

Directions:

1. First, you whisk eggs and cream/sour cream in a mixing bowl, until fluffy.
2. After which you add salt and pepper; add half of the shredded cheese and mix well.
3. After that, you melt the butter in a frying pan on medium heat; sauté the onion, diced ham and peppers for a few minutes.
4. Then you add the egg mixture and fry until the omelet is almost firm. (NOTE: Be extra mindful not to burn the edges).
5. Furthermore, you reduce the heat after a little while.
6. Finally, you sprinkle the rest of the cheese on top and fold the omelet.

7. Make sure you serve immediately... and enjoy!

Note:

Pair this recipe with a fresh, green salad. Feel free to serve with Tabasco or Sriracha sauce, or jalapenos on the side if you like to keep it spicy.

Low-carb ginger smoothie

Ingredients

2/3 cup of water

2 teaspoons of fresh ginger (grated)

1/3 cup of coconut milk (or better still coconut cream)

2 tablespoons of lime juice

1 oz. frozen spinach

Directions:

1. First, you mix all ingredients together; starting with 1 tablespoon lime and increase the amount to taste.
2. Then you sprinkle with some grated ginger and serve. So tasty!!

NOTE:

Meanwhile, you prepare your smoothies ahead of time to ease the morning rush. Make sure it last in the fridge for up to 2 days, using an airtight lid and remember to shake well before drinking!

Low-carb coconut cream with berries

Ingredients

2 oz. of fresh strawberries

1 pinch of vanilla extract

½ cup of coconut cream

Directions:

1. First, you mix all ingredients using an immersion blender.
2. Feel free to also add 1 teaspoon – 1 tablespoon of coconut oil to increase the fat ratio.

NOTE:

You can substitute strawberries for blueberries, raspberries or blackberries.

Scrambled eggs with basil and butter

Ingredients

2 tablespoons of coconut cream (or better still coconut milk or sour cream)

1 oz. butter

2 tablespoons of fresh basil

2 eggs

Salt

Shredded cheese (it is optional)

Directions:

1. First, you melt butter in a pan on low heat.
2. After which you mix together cream, eggs, and salt and add to the pan.
3. After that, you stir with a spatula from the edge towards the center until the eggs are scrambled. (NOTE: for me, I like it soft and creamy, not with a crisp surface, which means stirring often on lower heat).
4. Feel free to remove the pan from the heat when you add the batter; this is usually enough to keep the eggs soft.

Pancakes with berries and whipped cream

Ingredients

7 oz. cottage cheese

2 oz. butter (or better still coconut oil)

4 eggs

1 tablespoon of ground psyllium husk powder

Toppings

1 cup of heavy whipping cream

8 tablespoons of fresh raspberries (or better still fresh blueberries or fresh strawberries)

Directions:

1. First, you blend all ingredients for the batter in a bowl with a spoon or a big fork.
2. After which you let expand for 5 minutes or more.
3. After that, you heat butter or oil in a frying pan.
4. Then you fry the pancakes on medium heat for about 3–4 minutes on each side.
5. At this point, you flip very carefully (NOTE: be sure not to let the cottage cheese lumps stick to the pan as they melt).

6. Finally, you serve with blueberries or other berries, and heavy cream whipped until soft peaks form.

NOTE:

Remember, these pancakes are also a great snack served cold!

Frittata with fresh spinach

Ingredients

1 cup of heavy whipping cream

5 1/3 oz. diced bacon or better still chorizo

Salt and pepper

8 eggs

8 oz. of fresh spinach

5 1/3 oz. shredded cheese

2 tablespoons of butter (for frying)

Directions:

1. Meanwhile, you heat the oven to 350°F (175°C).
2. After which you fry the bacon in butter until crispy; add the spinach.
3. After that, you whisk the eggs and cream together and pour into a greased baking dish.
4. Then you add the spinach, bacon and cheese on top and place in the middle of the oven.
5. Then you bake for about 25–30 minutes.

NOTE:

I suggest you try this recipe with shredded green or red cabbage with a homemade dressing.

THE GLOW 15 COOKBOOK

Classic bacon and eggs

Ingredients

5 1/3 oz. bacon (in slices)

Fresh parsley (it is optional)

8 eggs

Cherry tomatoes (it is optional)

Directions:

1. First, you fry the bacon in a pan until crispy.
2. After which you put aside on a plate.
3. Then you fry the eggs in the bacon grease any way you like them.
4. At this point, you cut the cherry tomatoes in half and fry them at the same time.
5. Finally, you season with salt and pepper to taste.

NOTE:

I will suggest you step up your bacon game with organic bacon if you can find it... it is tastier and has fewer additives.

Laura's keto pancakes

Ingredients

2 eggs

1 teaspoon of maple extract

2 tablespoons of coconut oil (for frying)

2/3 oz. pork rinds

2 tablespoons of unsweetened cashew milk

1 teaspoon of ground cinnamon

Directions:

1. First, you place the pork rinds in a blender and pulse until ground into a fine powder.
2. After which you add the rest of the ingredients and combine until smooth.
3. After that, you heat a skillet to medium heat; once hot, add a tablespoon of coconut oil.
4. Then you pour ¼ cup batter into the skillet.
5. At this point, you fry until golden brown and set, about 2 minutes.
6. Furthermore, you flip and continue to cook until cooked all the way through.

7. Finally, you remove from skillet and repeat with remaining batter. Add more coconut oil as needed.

NOTE:

Feel free to add browned butter or a dollop of sour cream for a finishing touch. Also a few fresh raspberries add festive color and a tart but sweet finish.

Italian breakfast casserole

Ingredients

12 oz. of Italian sausage

8 eggs

5 oz. of shredded cheese

Salt and pepper

7 oz. of cauliflower

2 oz. butter

1 cup of heavy whipping cream

4 tablespoons of fresh basil

Directions:

1. Meanwhile, you heat the oven to 400°F (200°C).
2. After which you rinse and trim the cauliflower and chop into bite-sized pieces.
3. After that, you add butter to a skillet and fry the cauliflower over medium-high heat until it begins to soften.
4. Then you add sausage to the pan and use a spoon or spatula to break it up into crumbles.
5. Furthermore, you keep frying until the sausage is thoroughly cooked and the mixture is golden brown.

6. After which you season with salt and pepper to taste.
7. Then you grease a baking dish and add the sausage mixture.
8. At this point, you add all remaining ingredients except for the basil to a medium-sized bowl.
9. After that, you whisk to combine; season with salt and pepper.
10. This is when you pour the egg mixture over the sausage and add the basil on top.
11. Finally, you bake for about 30-40 minutes or until golden brown on top and completely set in the middle.
12. Remember, if the casserole is at risk of getting burned before it's cooked through, I suggest you cover with a piece of aluminum foil.

Note:

I suggest you try this dish with hot or mild Italian sausage. Or, better still mix it up with some of both!

Remember, if your sausage comes in links, I will suggest you just cut away the casing and sauté the loose ground meat.

Bacon and mushroom breakfast casserole

Ingredients

10 oz. bacon

8 eggs

5 oz. of shredded cheddar cheese

Salt and pepper

6 oz. of mushrooms

2 oz. butter

1 cup of heavy whipping cream

1 teaspoon of onion powder

Directions:

1. Meanwhile, you heat the oven to 400°F (200°C).
2. After which you trim the mushrooms and cut them in quarters.
3. After that, you dice the bacon; fry the bacon and mushrooms in butter in a skillet over medium-high heat until golden brown.
4. Then you season with salt and pepper to taste.
5. At this point, you place contents of the skillet in a greased baking dish.

6. After which you add remaining ingredients to a medium-sized bowl and whisk to combine.
7. Furthermore, you season with salt and pepper.
8. After that, you pour egg mixture over the bacon and mushrooms and bake in the oven for about 30-40 minutes or until golden brown on top and set in the middle.
9. Finally, you cover with a piece of aluminum foil if the top of the casserole is at risk of burning before it's cooked through.

NOTE:

Feel free to add spinach or other greens (to add a little color) to the skillet with the bacon and mushroom mixture in step 3 before frying, toward the end when almost finished cooking.

You can sauté for just a minute or two and proceed with the recipe.

Croque Monsieur

Ingredients

4 eggs

4 tablespoons of butter (or better still coconut oil for frying)

½ finely chopped red onion (it is optional)

8 oz. cottage cheese

1 tablespoon of ground psyllium husk powder

5 1/3 oz. smoked deli ham

5 1/3 oz. of cheddar cheese

<u>Directions for serving</u>

3½ oz. lettuce

4 tablespoons of olive oil

½ tablespoon of red wine vinegar

Salt and pepper

Directions:

1. First, you whisk the eggs in a bowl.
2. After which you mix in the cottage cheese.

3. After that, you add ground psyllium husk powder while stirring to incorporate it smoothly, without lumps.

4. Then you let the mixture rest for five minutes until the batter has set.

5. At this point, you place a frying pan over medium heat.

6. Furthermore, you add a generous amount of butter and fry the batter like small pancakes for a couple of minutes on each side, until they are golden.

7. After that, you make two pancakes per serving; assemble a sandwich with sliced ham and cheese between two of the warm pancakes.

8. Then you add finely chopped onion on top.

9. This is when you wash and tear the lettuce; mix vinegar, oil, salt and pepper into a simple vinaigrette.

10. Finally, you serve the Croque Monsieur warm beside lettuce dressed with the vinaigrette.

NOTE:

If you happen to put a fried egg on top and you'll have a Croque Madame!

Salami and Brie cheese plate

Ingredients

4 oz. of salami

1 avocado

4 tablespoons of olive oil

7 oz. Brie cheese

2 oz. lettuce

½ cup of macadamia nuts

Directions:

1. First, you put salami, avocado, cheese, lettuce, and nuts on a plate.
2. Then you drizzle oil over the salad and serve.

Note:

Remember that it doesn't have to be salami any fatty deli meat will do. Soppressata, pepperoni, coppa, or speck are all delicious substitutes, so feel free and use any of them!

Italian keto plate

Ingredients

7 oz. of prosciutto (sliced)

1/3 cup of olive oil

Salt and pepper

7 oz. of fresh mozzarella cheese

2 tomatoes

10 green olives

Directions:

1. First, you put prosciutto, tomatoes, cheese and olives on a plate.
2. Then you serve with olive oil and season with salt and pepper to taste.

NOTE:

Feel free to swap out the prosciutto for another fatty Italian deli meat.

Shrimp and artichoke plate

Ingredients

2/3 lb. of cooked and peeled shrimp

6 sun-dried tomatoes in oil

1½ oz. of baby spinach

Salt and pepper

4 eggs

14 oz. of canned artichokes

½ cup of mayonnaise

4 tablespoons of olive oil

Directions:

1. First, you begin by cooking the eggs.
2. After which you lower them carefully into boiling water and boil for about 4-8 minutes depending on whether you like them soft or hard boiled.
3. After that, you cool the eggs in ice-cold water for about 1-2 minutes when they're done; this will make it easier to remove the shell.
4. Then you place shrimp, mayonnaise, eggs, artichokes, sun-dried tomatoes and spinach on a plate.

5. Finally, you drizzle olive oil over the spinach. Season to taste with salt and pepper and serve.

NOTE:

For best flavor, I will suggest you buy your artichoke hearts and sun-dried tomatoes packed in olive oil.

Pesto chicken casserole with feta cheese and olives

Ingredients

2 oz. butter (for frying)

1½ cups of heavy whipping cream

8 oz. feta cheese (diced)

Salt and pepper

1½ lbs. of chicken thighs (or better still chicken breasts)

3 oz. of red pesto (or better still green pesto)

8 tablespoons of pitted olives

1 garlic clove (finely chopped)

Ingredients for serving:

4 tablespoons of olive oil

Sea salt and ground black pepper

5 1/3 oz. leafy greens

Directions:

1. Meanwhile, you heat the oven to 400°F (200°C).
2. After which you cut the chicken thighs or filets into pieces.

3. After that, you season with salt and pepper and fry in butter until golden brown.
4. Then you mix pesto and heavy cream in a bowl.
5. At this point, you place the fried chicken pieces in a baking dish together with olives, feta cheese and garlic; add the pesto.
6. Finally, you bake in oven for about 20-30 minutes, until the dish turns bubbly and light brown around the edges.

Caprese omelet

Ingredients

6 eggs

1 tablespoon of fresh basil (or dried basil)

Salt and pepper

2 tablespoons of olive oil

3½ oz. cherry tomatoes (cut in halves or tomatoes cut in slices)

5 1/3 oz. fresh mozzarella cheese

Directions:

1. First, you crack the eggs into a mixing bowl, add salt and black pepper to your liking.
2. After which you whisk well with a fork until fully combined; add basil and stir.
3. After that, you cut the tomatoes in halves or slices.
4. Then you dice or slice the cheese.
5. At this point, you heat oil in a large frying pan; fry the tomatoes for a few minutes.
6. Furthermore, you pour the egg batter on top of the tomatoes.

7. After that, you wait until the batter is slightly firm before adding the mozzarella cheese.
8. Finally, you lower the heat and let the omelet set.
9. Make sure you serve right away and enjoy!

Keto meat pie

Ingredients

1 garlic clove (finely chopped)

1 1/3 lbs. of ground beef (or better still ground lamb)

1 tablespoon of dried oregano (or better still dried basil)

½ cup of water

½ yellow onion (finely chopped)

2 tablespoons of butter (or better still olive oil)

Salt and pepper

4 tablespoons of tomato paste (or better still ayvar relish)

Ingredients Pie crust

4 tablespoons of sesame seeds

1 tablespoon of ground psyllium husk powder

1 pinch of salt

4 tablespoons of water

¾ cup of almond flour

4 tablespoons of coconut flour

1 teaspoon of baking powder

3 tablespoons of olive oil or coconut oil

1 egg

Topping

7 oz. shredded cheese

8 oz. cottage cheese

Directions:

1. Meanwhile, you heat the oven to 350°F (175°C).
2. After which you fry onion and garlic in butter or olive oil over medium heat for a few minutes, until the onion is soft.
3. After that, you add the ground beef and keep frying.
4. Then you add oregano or basil and add salt and pepper to taste.
5. At this point, you add tomato paste, pesto or ayvar relish (NOTE: use what you have on hand).
6. Furthermore, you add water; lower the heat and let simmer for at least 20 minutes.
7. After that, while the meat simmers, make the dough for the crust.
8. Then you mix all the dough ingredients in a food processor for a few minutes until the dough turns into a ball. (NOTE: if you don't have a food processor, you can mix by hand with a fork).
9. This is when you place a round piece of parchment paper in a well-greased spring form pan (about 10 inches in diameter) to make it easier to remove the pie when it's done. (NOTE: You can also use a deep-dish pie pan.)

10.   Spread the dough in the pan and up along the sides; use a spatula or well-greased fingers.

11. Meanwhile, you bake the crust for about 10-15 minutes.
12. After which, you take it out of the oven and place the meat in the crust.
13. After that, you mix cottage cheese and shredded cheese together, and layer on top of the pie.
14. Finally, you bake for about 30-40 minutes on lower rack or until the pie has turned a golden color.
15. Make sure you serve with a fresh green salad and dressing.

Glow Carbonara

Ingredients

1 tablespoon of butter

4 tablespoons of mayonnaise

Fresh parsley (chopped)

3 oz. grated parmesan cheese

2/3 lb. bacon or pancetta (diced)

1¼ cups of heavy whipping cream

Salt and pepper

2 lbs. of zucchini

4 egg yolks

Directions:

1. First, you pour the heavy cream into a saucepan and bring it to a boil.
2. After which you lower the heat and let boil for a few minutes until reduced by a fourth.
3. After that, you fry pancetta/bacon in butter until crispy (NOTE: reserve the fat).

4. Then you mix in the mayonnaise into the heavy cream.
5. At this point, you salt and pepper to taste, and cook until mayonnaise is warmed through.
6. This is when you make spirals of the zucchini with a spiralizer.

NOTE: if you don't have a spiralizer, I suggest you make thin zucchini strips with a potato peeler.

7. Furthermore, you add noodles to the warm cream sauce.
8. After which you divide between four plates and top with egg yolks, parsley, bacon, and a generous amount of freshly grated parmesan.
9. Finally, you drizzle bacon grease on top and serve immediately.

NOTE:

However, instead of adding raw noodles to the warm sauce, I suggest you also microwave the zucchini strands on high for a minute before topping them with sauce.

Glow no-noodle chicken soup

Ingredients

- 2 celery stalks
- 2 garlic cloves (minced)
- 2 teaspoons of dried parsley
- ¼ teaspoon of ground black pepper
- 1 medium-sized carrot
- 2 cups of green cabbage (sliced into strips)
- 4 oz. butter
- 6 oz. of sliced mushrooms
- 2 tablespoons of dried minced onion
- 1 teaspoon of salt
- 8 cups of chicken broth
- 1½ shredded rotisserie chickens

Directions:

1. First, you melt the butter in a large pot.
2. After which you slice the celery stalks and mushrooms into smaller pieces.

3. Then you add celery, dried onion, mushrooms and garlic into the pot and cook for three to four minutes.
4. At this point, you add carrot, salt, broth, parsley, and pepper.
5. After that, you simmer until vegetables are tender.
6. Finally, you add cooked chicken and cabbage; simmer for an additional 8 to 12 minutes until the cabbage "noodles" are tender.

Salad in a jar

Ingredients

1/6 oz. of leafy greens

1/6 oz. of red bell peppers

4 tablespoons of mayonnaise (or better still olive oil)

4 oz. smoked salmon or better still rotisserie chickens or other protein of your choice

1/6 oz. of cherry tomatoes

1/6 oz. of cucumber

½ scallion

Directions:

1. First, you shred or chop vegetables of your choice.
2. After which you put dark leafy greens such as spinach or arugula at the bottom of the jar (NOTE: iceberg lettuce or romaine works too, green and red cabbage gives a fresh crunch; chopped broccoli or cauliflower also works great).
3. After that, you add sliced shredded carrot, onion rings, avocado, different bell peppers and tomato in layers.
4. Then you top your salad with smoked salmon and grilled chicken, but you can of course use your own favorite protein,

mackerel, boiled eggs, or canned tuna fish or any kind of cold cuts you want (**NOTE:** Olives, seeds, nuts, and cheese cubes are great flavorful additions).

5. Remember if you want to feel satisfied, add a generous amount of dressing or mayonnaise that you store in a separate little jar or bottle and add right before serving.

Smoked salmon plate

Ingredients

1 cup of mayonnaise

1 tablespoon of olive oil

Salt and pepper

¾ lb. of smoked salmon

2 oz. of baby spinach

½ lime (it is optional)

Directions:

1. First, you put spinach, salmon, a wedge of lime, and a hearty dollop of mayonnaise on a plate.
2. Then you drizzle olive oil over the spinach and season with salt and pepper.

Note:

You can swap out the salmon for any fatty fish you enjoy. (NOTE: herring, sardines, Mackerel, and anchovies are all great options.) Feel free to also vary the greens—try shredded cabbage or spicy arugula.

Asian cabbage stir-fry
Ingredients

5 1/3 oz. butter

1 teaspoon of salt

¼ teaspoon of ground black pepper

2 garlic cloves

1 teaspoon of chili flakes

1 tablespoon of sesame oil

12⁄3 lbs. of green cabbage

11⁄3 lbs. of ground beef

1 teaspoon of onion powder

1 tablespoon of white wine vinegar

3 scallions (in slices)

1 tablespoon of fresh ginger (finely chopped or grated)

THE GLOW 15 COOKBOOK

Wasabi mayonnaise

½ - 1 tablespoon of wasabi paste

1 cup of mayonnaise

Directions:

1. First, you shred the cabbage finely using a sharp knife or a food processor.
2. After which you fry the cabbage in 2–3 ounces (about 60–90 g) butter in a large frying or wok pan on medium-high heat, but don't let the cabbage turn brown (NOTE: it takes a while for the cabbage to soften).
3. After that, you add spices and vinegar.
4. Then you stir and fry for a couple of minutes more.
5. At this point, you put the cabbage in a bowl.
6. After which you melt the rest of the butter in the same frying pan.
7. This is when you add garlic, chili flakes and ginger and sauté for a few minutes.
8. Furthermore, you add ground meat and brown until the meat is thoroughly cooked and most of the juices have evaporated; lower the heat a little.
9. After that, you add scallions and cabbage to the meat.
10. Then you stir until everything is hot.
11. Finally, you add salt and pepper to taste, and top with the sesame oil before serving; mix together the wasabi mayonnaise.

Glow quesadillas

Ingredients

Low-carb tortillas

2 egg whites

1½ teaspoons of ground psyllium husk powder

½ teaspoon of salt

2 eggs

6 oz. cream cheese

1 tablespoon of coconut flour

Filling

1 oz. leafy greens

1 tablespoon of olive oil (for frying)

5 oz. shredded cheese

Directions:

Tortillas

1. Meanwhile, you heat the oven to 400°F (200°C).
2. After which you beat the eggs and egg whites together until fluffy. (About 2-3 minutes with a mixer should do the trick.)

3. After that, you add the cream cheese and continue to beat until the batter is smooth.
4. Then you combine the psyllium husk powder, salt, and coconut flour in a small bowl and mix well.
5. At this point, you add this flour mixture one spoonful at a time into the batter while beating.
6. Furthermore, when combined, I suggest you let the batter sit for a few minutes.

NOTE: it should be as thick as pancake batter; your brand of psyllium husk powder affects this step — be patient... If it does not thicken enough, I will suggest you add more powder next time.

7. This is when you place parchment paper on two baking sheets.
8. After that, you pour three circles on each sheet, for a total of six tortillas.
9. Then you use a spatula to spread the batter into thin, ¼ inch thick rounds (NOTE: each tortilla should be about 5" across).
10. Finally, you bake on the upper rack for about 5 minutes (NOTE: the tortillas will turn a little brown around the edges when done). Make sure you keep your eye on the oven—don't let these tasty creations burn on the bottom!

Directions for the Quesadillas

1. First, you place three tortillas on a large cutting board.
2. After which you spoon half the grated cheese on the tortillas.
3. After that, you add a handful of leafy greens, sprinkle with remaining cheese, and top with another tortilla.
4. Then you heat a small, non-stick skillet; add oil (or butter) if desired.
5. At this point, you fry each quesadilla for about a minute on each side (NOTE: you'll know it's done when the cheese melts).

6. Finally, you cut quesadillas into wedges and serve.

Note:

Please, never underestimate the power of melted cheese—in other words, you should always make extra if you're expecting a crowd! And on the other hand make some guacamole, too.

Pork chops with green beans and garlic butter

Ingredients

2 oz. of butter (for frying)

Salt and pepper

4 pork chops

1 lb. of fresh green beans

Garlic butter

1 tablespoon of dried parsley

Salt and pepper

5 oz. butter (at room temperature)

½ tablespoon of garlic powder

1 tablespoon of lemon juice

Directions:

1. First, you take the butter out of the fridge and let it reach room temperature.
2. After which you mix garlic, butter, parsley and lemon juice.
3. After that, you season with salt and pepper to taste; set aside.
4. Then you make a few small cuts in the fat surrounding the chops to help them stay flat when frying.
5. At this point, you season with salt and pepper to taste.

6. After which you heat a frying pan over medium-high heat.
7. Furthermore, you add butter to the pan and add the chops; fry the chops for about 5 minutes on each side or until golden brown and thoroughly cooked through.
8. After that, you remove the chops from the pan and keep warm.
9. Then you use the same skillet and add the beans; season with salt and pepper to taste.
10. Finally, you cook over medium-high heat for a couple of minutes until the beans have a vibrant color and are slightly softened but still a bit crunchy.
11. Make sure you serve the pork chops and beans together with a dollop of garlic butter melting on top.

NOTE:

Remember that canned or frozen green beans may not be quite as crunchy, but still taste great and deliver easy nutrients straight from your freezer or pantry.

THE GLOW 15 COOKBOOK

Hamburger patties with creamy tomato sauce and fried cabbage

Ingredients

Hamburger Patties

1 egg

1 teaspoon of salt

2 oz. fresh parsley (finely chopped)

1/6 oz. butter

1½ lbs. of ground beef

3 oz. feta cheese

¼ teaspoon of ground black pepper

1 tablespoon of olive oil

Gravy

1 oz. fresh parsley (coarsely chopped)

Salt and pepper

¾ cup of heavy whipping cream

2 tablespoons of tomato paste (or better still ayvar relish)

Fried green cabbage

4¼ oz. butter

Salt and pepper

1½ lbs. of shredded green cabbage

Directions:

1. First, you mix all the ingredients for the hamburgers and form eight oblong patties.
2. After which you fry over medium-high heat in both butter and olive oil for at least 10 minutes or until the patties have turned a nice color.
3. After that, you pour the tomato paste and the whipping cream into the pan when the patties are almost done.
4. Then you stir and let the cream boil together; sprinkle chopped parsley on top before serving.
5. At this point, you butter-fried green cabbage.
6. This is when you shred the cabbage with a knife or use a food processor; melt butter in a frying pan.
7. Furthermore, you sauté the shredded cabbage over medium heat for at least 15 minutes or until the cabbage reaches desired color and consistency.
8. After that, you stir regularly and lower the heat a little towards the end.
9. Finally, you add salt and pepper to taste.

Roast beef and cheddar plate

Ingredients

5 oz. cheddar cheese

6 radishes

½ cup of mayonnaise

2 oz. lettuce

salt and pepper

7 oz. deli roast beef

1 avocado

1 scallion

1 tablespoon of Dijon mustard

2 tablespoons of olive oil

Directions:

1. First, you place cheese, roast beef, avocado and radishes on a plate.
2. After which you add sliced onion, mustard and a hearty dollop of mayonnaise.
3. Then you serve with lettuce and olive oil.

NOTE:

Feel free to swap out some of the mayo for butter, and try the radishes with butter and salt.

Glow chicken casserole

Ingredients

- 7 oz. shredded cheese
- ¾ lb. of cauliflower (in florets)
- 4 oz. cherry tomatoes
- ½ lemon (the juice)
- Salt and pepper
- 2 lbs. of chicken thighs
- 1 cup of heavy whipping cream
- 1 leek
- 2 tablespoons of green pesto
- 3 tablespoons of butter

Directions:

1. Meanwhile, you heat the oven to 400°F (200°C).
2. After which you mix cream (or sour cream) with pesto and lemon juice; salt and pepper to taste.
3. After that, you season the chicken thighs with salt and pepper, and fry in butter until they turn a nice golden brown.
4. Then you place the chicken in a baking dish, and pour in the cream mixture.
5. At this point, you chop the leek and cherry tomatoes.
6. Furthermore, you top chicken with leek, tomatoes and cauliflower.

7. Finally, you sprinkle cheese on top and bake in the middle of the oven for at least 30 minutes or until the chicken is fully cooked.

Glow shrimp and artichoke plate

Ingredients

2/3 lb. cooked and peeled shrimp

6 sun-dried tomatoes in oil4 eggs

½ cup mayonnaise

1½ oz. baby spinach

Salt and pepper

4 eggs

14 oz. canned artichokes

14 oz. canned artichokes

½ cup mayonnaise

4 tablespoons olive oil

Directions:

1. First, you begin by cooking the eggs.
2. After which you lower them carefully into boiling water and boil for about 4-8 minutes depending on whether you like them soft or hard boiled.
3. After that, you cool the eggs in ice-cold water for about 1-2 minutes when they're done; this will make it easier to remove the shell.
4. Then you place shrimp, mayonnaise, eggs, artichokes, sun-dried tomatoes and spinach on a plate.
5. At this point, you drizzle olive oil over the spinach.

6. Finally, you season to taste with salt and pepper and serve.

Note:

For best flavor, I suggest you buy your artichoke hearts and sun-dried tomatoes packed in olive oil.

Gingerbread crème brûlée

Ingredients

2 teaspoons of pumpkin pie spice

½ clementine (it is optional)

1¾ cups of heavy whipping cream

¼ teaspoon of vanilla extract

4 egg yolks

Directions:

1. Meanwhile, you heat the oven to 360°F (180°C).
2. After which you separate the eggs by cracking them and placing whites and yolks in separate bowls. (NOTE: this recipe only calls for yolks, so I will suggest you cover the egg white bowl with plastic wrap and store in the fridge for another recipe).
3. After that, you add cream to a saucepan and bring to a boil along with the spices and vanilla extract.
4. Then you add the warm cream mixture into the egg yolks, a little at a time, while whisking.
5. At this point, you pour into oven-proof ramekins or small Pyrex bowls nestled in a larger baking dish with sides.
6. Furthermore, you add water to the larger dish until it's about halfway up the ramekins. (NOTE: The water makes the cream cook gently and evenly for a creamy and smooth result).
7. After that, you bake in the oven for about 30 minutes.

8. Finally, you remove the ramekins from the baking dish and let cool.

9. Enjoy this dessert either lukewarm or cold, preferably with a clementine segment on top.

NOTE:

Use pumpkin pie spice in this recipe.

Then if you can't find it, I suggest you can make your own by using this recipe or by mixing equal amounts of cinnamon, ginger, and ground cloves.

Low-carb baked apples

Ingredients

1 oz. pecans (or walnuts)

½ teaspoon of ground cinnamon

1 tart/sour apple

2 oz. butter (at room temperature)

4 tablespoons of coconut flour

¼ teaspoon of vanilla extract

Ingredient for serving

½ teaspoon of vanilla extract

¾ cup of heavy whipping cream

Directions:

1. Meanwhile, you heat the oven to 350°F (175°C).
2. After which you mix chopped nuts, cinnamon, soft butter, coconut flour, and vanilla into a crumbly dough.
3. After that, you rinse the apple, but don't peel it or remove the seeds.
4. Then you cut off both ends and cut the middle part in four slices.
5. At this point, you place the slices in a greased baking dish and add dough crumbs on top.

6. Furthermore, you bake for about 15 minutes or more or until the crumbs turn golden brown.
7. After that, add heavy whipping cream and vanilla to a medium-sized bowl and whip until soft peaks form.
8. Finally, you let the apples cool for a couple of minutes and serve with a dollop of whipped cream.

NOTE:

Remember, these baked apples can be served with full-fat crème Fraiche, whipped cream, mascarpone, or a slice of cheddar.

If you're allergic to nuts you substitute sunflower or sesame seeds to keep the crunch.

Low-carb chocolate and peanut squares

Ingredients

4 tablespoons of butter (or coconut oil)

4 tablespoons of peanut butter

4 tablespoons of chopped salted peanuts (for decoration)

3½ oz. of dark chocolate with a minimum of 70% cocoa solids

1 pinch salt

½ teaspoon of vanilla extract

1 teaspoon of licorice powder or better still ground cinnamon or ground cardamom (green)

Directions:

1. First, you melt chocolate and butter or coconut oil in the microwave oven or in a double boiler.
2. (NOTE: If you don't have a double boiler you can put a glass bowl on top of a pot of steaming water, make sure that the water doesn't reach the bowl, the chocolate will melt from the heat of the steam).
3. After which you mix in all other ingredients and pour the batter into a small greased baking dish lined with parchment paper (no bigger than 4 x 6 inches).
4. After that, you let cool for a while and top with finely chopped peanuts or other creative toppings; refrigerate.

5. Finally, when the batter is set, cut into small squares with a sharp knife.

Note: keep these and all treats small -no more than a 1 x 1-inch square; make sure you store in the refrigerator or freezer.

NOTE:

Remember that almond or hazelnut butter work, too. Feel free to try different toppings: like toasted (and coarsely chopped) almonds or hazelnuts, roasted sesame seeds with unsweetened coconut flakes, or even tahini.

Low-carb chocolate fudge

Ingredients

1 teaspoon of vanilla extract

3 oz. dark chocolate with a minimum of 70% cocoa solids

2 cups of heavy whipping cream

3 oz. butter

Directions:

1. First, you boil heavy cream and vanilla in a heavy-bottomed saucepan.
2. After which you let it boil for a minute and lower the heat and simmer.
3. After that, you simmer the cream until it is reduced to half the amount – it will take about 20 minutes or more depending on how big the pan is and the temperature; stir occasionally.
4. Then you lower the heat and add room temperature butter.
5. At this point, you stir into a smooth batter; remove from heat.
6. Furthermore, you chop chocolate into small pieces.
7. After that, you add to the warm cream mixture and stir until the chocolate has melted; add additional flavorings if desired.
8. This is when you pour into a baking dish, about 7x7 inches (18 x 18 cm), and let cool in the refrigerator for a few hours.

9. Finally, you bring out and sprinkle cocoa powder on top; cut into pieces and serve cold.

10. Remember that this fudge can be kept in the freezer and doesn't need to be thawed; and it will be ready to enjoy after just a minute or two at room temperature.

NOTE:

Remember that this fudge is delicious as it is, but you can also add a flavor of your choice.

Feel free to try some licorice powder, instant coffee, peppermint oil or citrus zest; and if you're bold you can try a sprinkle of smoked chili or sea salt on top. Make sure you start with 1-2 teaspoons of flavoring when experimenting with the amount.

Low-carb coconut and chocolate pudding

Ingredients

2 egg yolks

1 teaspoon of vanilla extract

14 oz. coconut milk

3 oz. dark chocolate (with a minimum of 70% cocoa solids)

Directions:

1. First, you carefully bring coconut milk and egg yolks to a simmer, whisking continuously.
2. After which you let simmer while stirring for 10 minutes.
3. After that, you break the chocolate into a bowl.
4. Then you add the vanilla kernels and pour the coconut milk on top.
5. At this point, you let stand for a while so that the chocolate melts.
6. Finally, you whisk the batter together and pour into glasses; refrigerate for at least two hours before serving.

Low-carb blueberry ice cream

Ingredients

3 egg yolks

½ teaspoon of ground cardamom (green)

6 oz. blueberries (frozen)

1 cup of heavy whipping cream

½ teaspoon of vanilla extract

½ lemon (the zest)

8 oz. mascarpone cheese

Directions:

1. First, you take the blueberries from the freezer.
2. After which you whip the cream until soft peaks form and set aside.
3. After that, you beat egg yolks, vanilla, cardamom and lemon zest in a separate bowl until pale and fluffy.
4. Then you mix in the mascarpone cheese and then fold in the whipped cream.
5. Furthermore, you fold the half-thawed blueberries into the mixture.

6. At this point, you pour the mixture into a container with a lid and place in the freezer.
7. Finally, you stir the ice cream every 15 minutes until it firms up (NOTE: this takes about 1-1.5 hours).

Note:

You can substitute raspberries in place of blueberries for even fewer carbs, about 3.5 g per portion. Substitute cream cheese or ricotta for the mascarpone for a slightly different flavor profile.

Grilled peaches

Ingredients

2 tablespoons of butter (or better still coconut oil)

½ teaspoon of vanilla extract

3 ripe peaches

1 teaspoon of ground cinnamon

1 cup of heavy whipping cream

Directions:

1. First, you divide the peaches into four pieces and remove the pits.
2. After which you brush melted butter or oil on the cut surface and grill the wedges on an outdoor grill or in a grill pan NOTE: about a minute on each side will be enough).
3. Remember that you can also fry the peaches in a regular frying pan.
4. After that, you whisk the whipping cream to soft peaks and stir in the vanilla.
5. Then you powder cinnamon on top of the peaches and serve with the whipped cream.

NOTE:

You can serve the peaches with a generous amount of non-flavored Greek yogurt; and these grilled peaches adore a hint of vanilla or lime zest!

Low-carb coconut cream with berries

Ingredients

2 oz. fresh strawberries

1 pinch of vanilla extract

½ cup of coconut cream

Directions:

1. First, you mix all ingredients using an immersion blender.
2. Feel free to also add 1 teaspoon – 1 tablespoon of coconut oil to increase the fat ratio.

Note:

Strawberries can be substituted for raspberries, blueberries or blackberries.

Low-carb trifle

Ingredients

½ ripe banana

1 tablespoon of lime juice and some of the zest

2 oz. pecans (preferably roasted)

1 ripe avocado

¾ cup of coconut cream

1 tablespoon of vanilla extract

3 oz. fresh raspberries

Directions:

1. First, you mix together banana, avocado, coconut cream and half of the vanilla.
2. After which you mix the berries and the rest of the vanilla separately.
3. After that, you fill nice glasses or dessert bowls with alternating layers of the two mixtures.
4. Then you top with roasted nuts and serve as a dessert.

Note:

Feel free to add flavor to the coconut and avocado batter with some cinnamon, cardamom or perhaps cocoa and coffee powder.

Remember that this trifle creates the perfect backdrop for tons of sweet and savory combinations!

Make sure you serve in a clear glass for a gorgeous presentation.

Brussels sprouts with caramelized red onions

Ingredients

1 red onion

Salt and pepper

4¼ oz. butter

1 tablespoon of red wine vinegar

1 lb. Brussels sprouts

Directions:

1. First, you divide the onions into wedges and fry in butter on medium heat for 5–10 minute.
2. Remember, the onions should turn golden, but not burned.
3. After which you add the vinegar and season with salt and pepper to taste.
4. After which you lower the heat some and continue to sauté the onion while stirring; place on a plate.
5. Then you cut the Brussels sprouts in half, depending on their size (NOTE: if they are small, fry them whole).
6. At this point, you fry the Brussels sprouts in the same frying pan with more butter until they have turned a nice color and a little soft.
7. Furthermore, you use a knife or a pin to check (NOTE: They're best served "al dente").
8. Finally, you salt and pepper; then add the onions and stir.

Green beans with roasted onions and cream of mushroom sauce

Ingredients

½ teaspoon salt

2 tablespoons coconut flour

Cream of mushroom sauce

1/6 oz. butter

½ teaspoon of onion powder

½ teaspoon of pepper

½ tablespoon of Dijon mustard

1 yellow onion

½ teaspoon of onion powder

1 1/3 lbs. fresh green beans

5 1/3 oz. mushrooms (or preferably other mixed mushrooms)

2/3 cup of heavy whipping cream

½ teaspoon of garlic powder

1 tablespoon of dried chives

½ tablespoon of tamari soy sauce (it is optional)

Directions:

1. Meanwhile, you heat oven to 450°F (225°C).

2. After which you begin with the mushroom sauce; cut the mushrooms and slice or chop finely.

3. After that, you heat up the butter in a frying pan and brown quickly on high heat.

4. Then you let the mushrooms cook until they turn a light golden color.

5. At this point, you add spices, cream and optional mustard or soy sauce; let it simmer on medium heat for about 10-15 minutes.

6. After which you stir occasionally; season with salt and pepper.

7. Furthermore, you remove from the stove and cool slightly.

8. After that, you puree in a blender or food processor (or use a hand blender in a deep bowl), until the consistency is smooth and creamy.

9. Then you dilute with more cream until sauce has the desired consistency.

10. This is when you cut the onion in thin rings and put them in a plastic bag.

11. This is the point, you pour in powdered onion, salt, and coconut flour; shake until onion rings are evenly coated.

12. After that, you spread the rings on a baking sheet covered with parchment paper and drizzle lightly with olive oil.

13. Then you roast onions in the oven for roughly 15 minutes (NOTE: they brown quickly at the end, so keep a close eye on them and remove from oven before they burn).

14. Make sure you chop the ends off the beans and slice them lengthwise down the middle.

15. Then blanch in plenty of lightly salted water for a few minutes; they should be bright green.

16. Finally, you pour the cream of mushroom sauce over them and top the dish with the onion rings.

Roasted tomato salad

Ingredients

- 1 lb. cherry tomatoes
- ½ teaspoon of ground black pepper
- 1 tablespoon of red wine vinegar
- 3 tablespoons of olive oil
- 1 teaspoon of sea salt
- ½ cup of finely chopped scallions

Directions:

1. First, you brush the tomatoes with oil to cover and sprinkle with spices.
2. After which cook on the grill, using a special vegetable accessory, or in the oven until the tomatoes have browned a bit.

NOTE: if using the oven, I suggest you bake at 450°F (225°C) for about 15 minutes.

3. After that, you stir and turn the oven off, but leave the tomatoes to bake a little longer about 10 more minutes.
4. Then you plate and sprinkle chopped scallions on top.
5. Furthermore, you drizzle with vinegar and the rest of the olive oil.
6. Finally, you let rest so the flavors mingle; serve the salad lukewarm or cold.

Note:

You can chop the tomatoes in rough pieces if you prefer a more salsa-like salad. Or, better still throw on some crumbled feta for extra flavor.

Butter-fried kale with pork and cranberries

Ingredients

> 1 lb. kale
>
> ½ cup of frozen cranberries
>
> 3 oz. butter
>
> ¾ lb. of smoked pork belly or bacon
>
> 2 oz. pecans (or better still walnuts)

Directions:

1. First, you rinse, trim and chop kale into large chunks; set aside.
2. After which you cut the pork belly into strips (or preferably use strips of bacon) and fry in butter over medium-high heat until golden brown and crispy.
3. After that, you add kale to the pan and fry for a couple of minutes until wilted.
4. Then you turn off the heat and add cranberries and nuts to the pan and stir.
5. Make sure you serve immediately.

Note:

This tasty recipe can easily be made into an entire meal by adding a couple of fried eggs. For variety, I suggest you try substituting kale for Tuscan cabbage or fresh spinach.

Low-carb cauliflower mash

Ingredients

3 oz. grated parmesan cheese

Olive oil (it is optional)

1 lb. cauliflower

4 oz. butter

½ lemon (juice and zest)

Directions:

1. First, you cut the cauliflower into florets.
2. After which you boil the cauliflower in plenty of lightly salted water a couple of minutes – just enough so the florets are tender but retain a somewhat firm texture.
3. After that, you discard the water.
4. Then you blend with the other ingredients in a food processor or use a hand blender.
5. Furthermore, you season with salt and pepper to taste.
6. Finally, you add more olive oil or butter if you wish.

Note:

There are colorful varieties of cauliflower available, but I suggest you stick to the white for the best mashing potential. You can also use pre-packaged "riced" cauliflower, if you don't have a fresh cauliflower.

Low-carb cauliflower cheese

Ingredients

1 cup of heavy whipping cream

Salt and pepper

7 oz. cream cheese

2 teaspoons of garlic powder

1 lb. broccoli (frozen or fresh)

2 oz. butter

1¾ lbs. cauliflower

2 cups of shredded cheese

Directions:

1. First, you set the oven to 350°F (180°C).
2. After which you boil the broccoli until it is fork tender.
3. Then, when done, strain and discard the water.
4. After that, you add cream cheese, salt, heavy whipping cream, pepper and garlic powder.
5. At this point, you puree with a hand blender until smooth.
6. This is when you grease a baking dish with butter and place the rest of the butter in pieces in the baking dish.
7. Furthermore, you cut the cauliflower into small florets and add to the baking dish.
8. Then you pour the broccoli cream sauce over the florets and top with shredded cheese.

9. Finally, you bake in oven for about 40 minutes or until the cauliflower is fork-tender and the top is golden brown.

Note:

If you are a vegetarian, I suggest you enjoy this dish with a couple of egg.

Butter-roasted cauliflower

Ingredients

5 1/3 oz. butter

Salt and pepper

2 lbs. cauliflower

Directions:

1. Meanwhile, you heat the oven to 400°F (200°C).
2. After which you trim and cut the cauliflower into small florets; the smaller, the quicker they will be done.
3. After that, you place in a large baking dish; salt and pepper to taste.
4. Then you cover with thin slices of butter.
5. Finally, you bake on upper rack in the oven and roast for about 20 minutes or more, depending on size of the florets.

Red coleslaw

Ingredients

1¼ cups of mayonnaise

¼ teaspoon of ground black pepper

1 tablespoon of whole-grain mustard

12/3 lbs. red cabbage

1 teaspoon of salt

2 teaspoons of ground caraway seeds

Directions:

1. First, you shred the cabbage finely, with a mandolin slicer or in a food processor.
2. After which you mix with other ingredients and let sit for about 10–15 minutes before serving.

Note:

If you have leftover shredded cabbage, I suggest you refrigerate it in a tightly closed plastic bag for several days to use for another recipe... perhaps a crack slaw?

Glow zucchini fries with spicy tomato mayo

Ingredients

Zucchini Fries

1 cup of almond flour

1 teaspoon of onion powder

3 tablespoons of olive oil

2 lbs. zucchini

1 cup of grated parmesan cheese

½ teaspoon of ground black pepper

2 eggs

Spicy Tomato Mayo

1 teaspoon of tomato paste

Salt and ground black pepper (to taste)

1 cup of mayonnaise

½ teaspoon of Tabasco (or better still cayenne pepper)

Directions:

1. First, you mix together the ingredients for the tomato mayo and refrigerate.
2. Meanwhile, you heat the oven to 400°F (200°C).
3. After which you line a baking sheet with parchment paper.
4. After that, you crack the eggs into a shallow bowl and whisk until smooth.
5. Then you mix almond flour, parmesan cheese and spices in another bowl.
6. At this point, you cut the zucchini into sticks; remove the seeds (or better still leave them—your choice).
7. Furthermore, you dredge the zucchini sticks in the almond flour mixture until they are completely covered.
8. After that, you dip them in the egg batter and then again in the almond flour mixture.
9. Then you place the zucchini sticks on the baking sheet and drizzle on the olive oil.
10. Finally, you bake in the oven for about 20-25 minutes or until the fries have browned nicely.
11. Make sure you serve with the spicy tomato mayo.

NOTE:

You are free to open your mind to all the veggie fry possibilities… green beans, asparagus, and wax beans are yummy options.

Mango, Chili, and Lime Quinoa Salad [Vegan, Gluten-Free]

Ingredients

Zest and juice of 1/2 -1 lime (depending on size)

½ -1 green chili (depending on spice preference)

Handful of golden raisins

1 teaspoon of extra virgin olive oil

Handful of pecans and pumpkin seeds

¼ cup of quinoa (plus water for cooking)

¼ red onion

½ mango

1/3 red bell pepper

Lamb's lettuce

Directions:

1. First, you cook the quinoa and leave the saucepan with the lid on to fluff up until cool.
2. Then, while the quinoa is cooking zest and juice the lime into a bowl.
3. After, you slice the chili, onion, and mango then add to the lime juice with the golden raisins, stir, and leave to soak.
4. Furthermore, once the quinoa has cooled cut up the pepper and mix into the quinoa with the olive oil and lamb's lettuce then season with salt and pepper.

5.   Finally, you stir the soaked ingredients to the quinoa mixture, serve in a bowl and top with pecans and pumpkin seeds.

Blue Spirulina Smoothie Bowl [Vegan, Gluten-Free]

Ingredients

1 fresh banana (for stars and blending)

Vegan yogurt of choice (for topping)

Coconut flakes (for topping)

2 frozen bananas

1 tablespoon of agave nectar

3 or more blue spirulina capsules

Blackberries (for topping)

Directions:

1.   First, you slice a couple pieces of fresh banana and use a cookie cutter to make stars out of them.
2.   After which you process leftover frozen bananas, banana, and agave nectar in a food processor.
3.   Then, once smooth, empty spirulina caps and process more.
4.   At this point, you pour blue banana ice cream into a bowl.
5.   Finally, you add vegan yogurt, blackberries, banana stars, and coconut flakes.

Tropical Turmeric Smoothie [Vegan]

Ingredients

1 fresh banana

2 dates (pitted)

Water (for blending)

1 orange (peeled)

1 cup of frozen mango

1 thumb-sized turmeric (peeled)

Preparation

First, you blend all ingredients until smooth; only add a little water as needed for blending.

Notes

Make sure you add non-dairy milk or coconut butter for extra creaminess.

Cauliflower Brazil nut Purée with Crispy Tofu [Vegan]

Serves2

Ingredients

- 2 garlic cloves
- 4 Brazil nuts
- 1 teaspoon of sea salt
- 3/4 cup of extra firm tofu (cubed)
- 1 small head cauliflower (stems removed, cut into florets)
- 1 teaspoon of dried thyme
- 3 leaves Swiss chard (coarsely chopped)
- 1 teaspoon of freshly ground pepper
- 2 teaspoons of coconut oil (divided)

Directions:

1. First, you bring 2 cups water to a boil in a covered pot with a pinch of salt.
2. After which you add garlic, Brazil nuts, cauliflower, thyme, and chard and bring everything to a boil for 3 minutes.
3. Then, while it's coming to a boil, heat 1 teaspoon coconut oil in a skillet until glistening, then add tofu and cook until browned on each side.

4. At this point, you drain cauliflower pot, reserving ½ cup of the cooking liquid in a measuring cup.

5. Furthermore, you transfer cauliflower and everything else in the pot to a food processor.

6. After that, you add reserved cooking liquid and remaining teaspoon of coconut oil.

7. After which you blend until smooth.

8. Finally, you transfer purée to serving dishes and top with browned tofu.

Raw Portobello Burgers with Collard Greens and Guacamole
[Vegan, Gluten-Free]

Serves 2

Ingredients

Ingredients for the Burgers:

1 teaspoon of Bragg's liquid aminos or preferably tamari

¼ cup of sun-dried tomatoes

2 tablespoons of tahini

2 Portobello mushroom tops

1 cup of baby spinach leaves

2 huge collard leaves

Ingredients for the Guacamole:

1 tablespoon of lemon juice

1/8 teaspoon of chili flakes (it is optional)

1 avocado

¼ teaspoon of sea salt

¼ teaspoon of black pepper

Directions:

1. First, you toss the mushroom tops in the Bragg's or tamari.
2. After which you set in the dehydrator at 115 degrees (Fahrenheit) – or in your oven at its lowest temperature for about 30 minutes or until they soften and darken a little.

Directions on how to make the guacamole:

1. First, you mash the avocado flesh with the salt, lime juice, pepper and chili (if using).
2. After which you adjust according to taste (NOTE: some garlic might be nice).
3. After that, you take a mushroom top and spread on some guacamole, then pile with greens and tomatoes.
4. Finally, you drizzle in a little tahini if you like, then wrap up in a collard leaf!

Smoky Tomato Almond Pasta Sauce [Vegan]

Serves 2

Ingredients

1 small yellow onion (diced)

1 roasted red pepper (roughly chopped)

3 tablespoons of fresh parsley

A pinch of red chili flakes

1 13.5-ounce can fire roasted tomatoes

Ground almonds (for topping)

2 tablespoons of extra virgin olive oil

3 cloves garlic (minced)

½ cup of almond meal (ground almonds)

1 teaspoon of smoked paprika (or better still regular paprika)

¼ teaspoon of salt

Pasta of choice for 2

Directions:

1. First, you heat olive oil in a small saucepan over medium heat.

2. After which you add in onions and garlic and sauté until soft.

3. After that, you add roasted ground almonds, paprika, red pepper, parsley, chili, and salt and stir to combine. The mixture will look like a paste.

4. Then you continue to cook over medium heat, stirring often, for about 5-6 minutes until the almonds are fragrant and toasty.

5. At this point, you remove from heat and let cool.

6. Furthermore, you add mixture to a blender with tomatoes and blend until smooth, adding a drizzle of olive oil, if needed.

7. After that, you return the smooth sauce to a saucepan and simmer until pasta is ready, taste and adjust seasoning if needed.

8. Then you cook pasta according to package instructions.

9. Finally, you add a bit of the starchy pasta water to thin out the sauce towards the end of cooking, if needed.

10. Make sure you serve with a little extra fresh ground almond, parsley, and a drizzle of olive oil.

Chocolate Coconut Milk Mousse Recipe

Yield: 10 servings

Ingredients

4 tablespoons of cocoa or better still cacao powder

2 teaspoons of vanilla extract

3.5 oz. /100g chocolate (it is optional but delicious)

2 cans of coconut milk (not low-fat 400ml cans)

4 tablespoons of sweetener maple syrup (or coconut nectar or preferably any liquid sweetener)

A pinch of salt

Directions:

1. First, you shake the coconut milk and open the tins.
2. After which you pour into a bowl and whisk until it's all combined.
3. After that, you add the salt, cocoa or cacao, vanilla and whisk while adding the sweetener.
4. Then you whisk for 1 min with an electric whisk or about 2-3 mins with a manual whisk until it starts to thicken a bit.
5. At this point, you scrape the sides halfway through to ensure everything gets combined.
6. Remember, it will still be pourable, but will set in the fridge.

7. Furthermore, you pour into your serving dishes and place in the fridge for at least two hours.
8. Finally, you finely chop the chocolate, sprinkle on top and serve.

NOTE: the mousse will last a few days in the fridge.

Fruity Summer Rolls with Salted Caramel Dip Recipe

Yield: 10 rolls

Ingredients

About 10 Rice paper wraps

Fruit ingredients:

1/8th Watermelon

2 Kiwi fruits

20 Raspberries

1 Mango

2 Avocados

3 Bananas

2 Nectarines

20 Mint leaves

Salted caramel dip ingredients

1 cup or 100g dates

1 teaspoon of sea salt or pink salt

1 cup or 150g cashews

1 teaspoon of vanilla

Directions:

1. First, you chop all fruit into thin strips, apart from small fruit like berries and the mint leaves.
2. After which you submerge the rice paper in warm water for a few seconds, make sure you take out while it still has some shape as it will continue to soften once taken out of the water.
3. After that, you place rice paper flat on a flat surface and then add thin slices of fruit on 1/3 of the paper at an edge.
4. Then you roll the rice paper up by folding over the filling, tucking in the sides then rolling to the edge.
5. At this point, you add all of the salted caramel dip ingredients to a blender and add enough warm water to cover everything.
6. Furthermore, you blend until smooth, you may need to add more water if the blender can't break up everything / or if the dip is too stiff.
7. Finally, you slice all of the rolls in the middle and enjoy by dipping in the sauce.
8. Remember that they will last a few days in the fridge but are best eaten as soon as made.

CONCLUSION

These healthy recipes would help you Shred the Fat Instantly and keep the weight off for good.

If you follow religiously to some of the recipes outlined in this book. In just 15 days, you'll begin to harness the power of autophagy to drop pounds, get glowing skin, and restore your energy through, because it is proven to work.

Get in shape this Season taking this Delectable recipe.

CPSIA information can be obtained
at www.ICGtesting.com
Printed in the USA
BVHW011945220621
610234BV00012B/401